Active
Aging

Comprehensive Exercises
for Seniors

Bolakale Aremu
Ojula Technology Innovations

Limit of Liability/Disclaimer of Warranty

The information provided in this health and fitness book is for educational and informational purposes only. It is not intended to be a substitute for professional medical advice, diagnosis, or treatment. Always seek the advice of your physician or other qualified healthcare provider before beginning any new exercise program or making changes to your diet.

The author and publisher of this book have made every effort to ensure the accuracy and completeness of the information contained herein. However, they make no warranty, express or implied, with respect to the information provided in this book, including any warranties of fitness for a particular purpose.

The author and publisher shall not be liable for any loss, injury, or damages arising from the use or inability to use the information contained in this book, whether direct, indirect, special, incidental, or consequential, even if advised of the possibility of such damages.

By reading this book, you acknowledge that you have read this disclaimer and understand that the author and publisher are not responsible for any consequences that may arise from the use of the information contained herein.

Table of Contents

1. Introduction 9

    1.1. Definition of Active Aging................................9

    1.2. The Importance of Exercise for Seniors 11

    1.3. Benefits of Regular Exercise for Seniors.........13

    1.4. Overview of the Book.....................................14

2. Exercises for Seniors...17

    2.1. Types of Exercises Suitable for Seniors 17

    2.2. Factors to Consider Before Starting an Exercise
Program 18

    2.3. How to Get Started with an Exercise Program 20

    2.4. Common Exercise Mistakes to Avoid 21

3. Chair Exercises for Seniors 24

    3.1. Benefits of Chair Exercises 24

    3.2. Chair Exercises for the Upper Body...............25

    3.3. Chair Exercises for the Lower Body 26

    3.4. Chair Exercises for Flexibility and Balance 28

4. Balance Exercises for Seniors 30

4.1. The Importance of Balance Exercises for
Seniors 30

4.2. Balance Exercises for the Lower Body 31

4.3. Balance Exercises for the Upper Body.............33

4.4. Balance Exercises for Overall Balance and
Stability...34

5. Strength Training Exercises for Seniors..................37

5.1. Benefits of Strength Training for Seniors........37

5.2. Strength Training Exercises for the Upper Body
....38

5.3. Strength Training Exercises for the Lower Body
....39

5.4. How to Progress with Strength Training
Exercises 41

6. Low-Impact Cardio Exercises for Seniors 43

6.1. Benefits of Low-impact Cardio Exercises.......43

6.2. Low-impact Cardio Exercises for the Upper
Body...45

6.3. Low-impact Cardio Exercises for the Lower
Body...46

6.4. How to Progress with Low-impact Cardio
Exercises 47

7. Stretching Exercises for Seniors.............................50

7.1. Benefits of Stretching for Seniors....................50

7.2. Stretching Exercises for the Upper Body 51

7.3. Stretching Exercises for the Lower Body........52

7.4. How to Progress with Stretching Exercises.....54

8. Water Aerobics Exercises for Seniors.....................56

8.1. Benefits of Water Aerobics for Seniors...........56

8.2. Water Aerobics Exercises for the Upper Body57

8.3. Water Aerobics Exercises for the Lower Body
....58

8.4. How to Progress with Water Aerobics Exercises
....60

9. Yoga Exercises for Seniors 62

9.1. Benefits of Yoga for Seniors 62

9.2. Yoga Poses for Flexibility and Balance...........63

9.3. Yoga Poses for Strength and Endurance 65

9.4. How to Progress with Yoga Exercises.............66

10. Conclusion..69

10.1. Recap of the Benefits of Exercise for Seniors
....69

10.2. Encouragement to Continue an Active Lifestyle 70

10.3. Additional Resources for Seniors to Stay Active 72

10.4 Thank You! 75

1. Introduction

1.1. Definition of Active Aging

Active aging refers to the process of optimizing opportunities for health, participation, and security in order to enhance quality of life as people age. It involves staying physically and mentally active, engaging in social activities, and maintaining a healthy lifestyle.

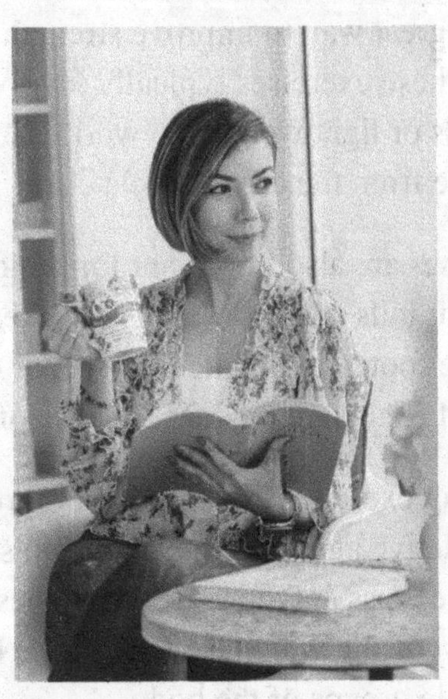

There are many benefits to active aging, including increased longevity, improved physical and mental health, and a greater sense of purpose and fulfillment. Older adults who remain active and engaged in life tend to have better cognitive function, stronger immune systems, and fewer chronic health conditions.

Exercise is a key component of active aging, and there are many different types of exercises that seniors can participate in to stay healthy and fit. Chair exercises, for example, are a great way to improve strength and flexibility while seated. These exercises typically involve using resistance bands or light weights to work the upper body, and can be done from the comfort of a chair.

Balance exercises are also important for seniors, as they can help prevent falls and injuries. These exercises involve standing on one foot, walking heel-to-toe, or other movements that challenge the body's sense of balance.

Strength training exercises are another important component of active aging, as they can help seniors maintain muscle mass and bone density. These exercises typically involve using weights or resistance bands to work the major muscle groups of the body.

Low-impact cardio exercises, such as walking, cycling, or swimming, are also great for seniors who want to stay active and maintain their cardiovascular health. These exercises are gentle on the joints and can be done at a low intensity to minimize the risk of injury.

Stretching exercises are important for maintaining flexibility and preventing muscle stiffness and soreness. These exercises can be done at home or in a group setting, and can help seniors feel more relaxed and comfortable in their bodies.

Water aerobics and yoga are also great options for seniors who want to stay active and engaged in life. These exercises provide a low-impact, full-body workout that can improve strength, balance, and flexibility, while also promoting relaxation and stress relief.

In summary, active aging is all about staying engaged in life and maintaining a healthy lifestyle as we age. Exercise is a key component of active aging, and there are many different types of exercises that seniors can participate in to stay healthy, fit, and happy. Whether you prefer chair exercises, balance exercises, strength training, low-impact cardio, stretching, water aerobics, or yoga, there is an exercise program out there that can help you stay active and engaged in life as you age.

1.2. The Importance of Exercise for Seniors

The importance of exercise for seniors cannot be overstated. As we age, it becomes increasingly important to maintain our physical health to ensure that we can continue to live an active and independent lifestyle. Exercise has been shown to have numerous benefits for seniors, including improving balance, strength, flexibility, and cardiovascular health.

One of the most important benefits of exercise for seniors is improved balance. As we age, our balance can deteriorate, which can increase the risk of falls and other injuries. Balance exercises, such as standing on one leg or walking heel-to-toe, can help seniors to improve their balance and reduce their risk of falls.

Strength training exercises are also important for seniors, as they can help to maintain muscle mass and prevent the loss of bone density. Strength training exercises can be done using weights or resistance bands, or even just using body weight exercises such as squats and push-ups.

Low-impact cardio exercises, such as walking, swimming, or cycling, can help seniors to maintain their cardiovascular health without putting too much stress on their joints. These exercises can help to improve circulation and reduce the risk of heart disease and other cardiovascular conditions.

Stretching exercises are also important for seniors, as they can help to improve flexibility and reduce the risk of injury. Yoga exercises are a particularly good option for seniors, as they can help to improve balance, strength, and flexibility all at once.

Finally, water aerobics exercises can be a great option for seniors who want to get some exercise while also taking the pressure off their joints. Water aerobics can help to improve cardiovascular health, strength, and flexibility, all while being easy on the joints.

In conclusion, exercise is incredibly important for seniors, and there are many different types of exercises that can be done to improve physical health. Whether it is chair exercises, balance exercises, strength training exercises, low-impact cardio exercises, stretching exercises, water aerobics exercises, or yoga exercises, there is something for everyone. By incorporating exercise into your daily routine, you can help to maintain your physical health and continue to live an active and independent lifestyle well into your senior years.

1.3. Benefits of Regular Exercise for Seniors

As we grow older, we tend to slow down and become less active. This can lead to a variety of health problems, including weight gain, weaker bones and muscles, and an increased risk of chronic diseases. But, by incorporating regular exercise into your daily routine, seniors can reap many benefits that improve overall health and quality of life.

One of the most significant benefits of regular exercise for seniors is its ability to improve balance and coordination. As we age, our balance can become compromised, and we become more prone to falls. However, by engaging in balance exercises such as standing on one foot or practicing yoga poses, seniors can improve their balance, reduce the risk of falls, and increase confidence in their movements.

Strength training exercises are also essential for seniors as they help build and maintain muscle mass. This, in turn, can improve overall strength, flexibility, and mobility, making everyday activities easier and reducing the risk of injuries. Chair exercises are a great option for those with limited mobility or those who prefer to exercise in a seated position.

Low-impact cardio exercises such as walking, cycling, or swimming are also beneficial for seniors. They help improve cardiovascular health, increase stamina, and boost mood and energy levels. Water aerobics exercises are a great low-impact option for those with joint problems, as the buoyancy of the water reduces the impact on joints.

Stretching exercises are also critical for seniors, as they help maintain flexibility and range of motion. Stretching can also improve posture, reduce stiffness and pain, and promote relaxation and stress reduction.

Overall, regular exercise for seniors offers numerous benefits that can improve quality of life and overall health. Whether it's through chair exercises, balance exercises, strength training, low-impact cardio, stretching, water aerobics, or yoga, there's an exercise for every senior to enjoy and benefit from. So, get moving and enjoy the many benefits of an active aging lifestyle!

1.4. Overview of the Book

Active Aging: Comprehensive Exercises for Seniors is a comprehensive guide that provides seniors with a range of exercises to help improve their physical and mental well-being. The book is specially designed for seniors who want to remain active and healthy, but are not sure where to start.

This book covers a wide range of exercises that are specifically designed for seniors. The exercises are divided into different categories, including chair exercises, balance exercises, strength training exercises, low-impact cardio exercises, stretching exercises, water aerobics exercises, and yoga exercises.

The chair exercises are perfect for seniors who have mobility issues or limited range of motion. These exercises are designed to be performed while seated and can help improve flexibility, strength, and balance.

The balance exercises are specifically designed to help improve balance and reduce the risk of falls. These exercises are particularly important for seniors who may have balance issues.

The strength training exercises are designed to help seniors build and maintain muscle mass. These exercises are important as they can help increase bone density and reduce the risk of sarcopenia.

The low-impact cardio exercises are perfect for seniors who want to improve their cardiovascular health without putting too much strain on their joints. These exercises can help improve endurance and overall health.

The stretching exercises are designed to help seniors improve their flexibility and reduce the risk of injury. These exercises can also help seniors relax and reduce stress.

The water aerobics exercises are perfect for seniors who want to exercise in a low-impact environment. These exercises can help improve cardiovascular health and overall fitness.

The yoga exercises are designed to help seniors improve their flexibility, strength, and balance. These exercises can also help seniors reduce stress and improve mental well-being.

In conclusion, Active Aging: Comprehensive Exercises for Seniors is an essential guide for seniors who want to remain active and healthy. With a range of exercises to choose from, seniors can improve their physical and mental well-being while enjoying the benefits of exercise.

2. Exercises for Seniors

2.1. Types of Exercises Suitable for Seniors

As we age, it is important to maintain an active lifestyle to help us stay healthy and independent. There are numerous types of exercises that are suitable for seniors, and each offers unique benefits that can help keep our bodies and minds in shape.

Chair exercises are a great option for seniors who may have difficulty standing or moving around. These exercises can be done while seated in a chair and can help improve flexibility, strength, and balance.

Balance exercises are important for seniors as they can help prevent falls and improve overall stability. Simple exercises like standing on one foot or walking heel-to-toe can help improve balance and coordination.

Strength training exercises are another important part of a senior's exercise routine. These exercises can include lifting weights or using resistance bands and can help improve muscle strength and bone density.

Low-impact cardio exercises like walking, swimming, or cycling can help improve cardiovascular health and overall endurance. These exercises are gentle on the joints and can be done at a pace that is comfortable for each individual.

Stretching exercises are important for seniors as they can help improve flexibility and range of motion. Simple stretches like reaching for the toes or stretching the arms and legs can help keep muscles limber and prevent injury.

Water aerobics exercises are a great option for seniors who may have joint pain or limited mobility. These exercises can be done in a pool and can help improve cardiovascular health and overall strength.

Yoga exercises are another great option for seniors as they can help improve flexibility, balance, and strength. Yoga can also be beneficial for mental health as it can help reduce stress and improve overall well-being.

In conclusion, there are many types of exercises that are suitable for seniors, and it is important to find the ones that work best for each individual. Incorporating a variety of exercises into a daily routine can help seniors stay healthy, active, and independent.

2.2. Factors to Consider Before Starting an Exercise Program

Starting an exercise program can be a daunting task, especially for seniors who are not used to exercising regularly. However, regular exercise can provide numerous benefits for seniors, including improved physical and mental health, increased energy levels, and better overall quality of life.

Before starting an exercise program, there are several factors that seniors should consider to ensure they are exercising safely and effectively. These factors include:

1. Health status: Seniors should consider their overall health status before starting an exercise program. They should consult with their healthcare provider to determine if there are any health concerns or conditions that may affect their ability to exercise.

2. Fitness level: Seniors should also consider their current fitness level and choose exercises that are appropriate for their level of fitness. It is important to start slowly and gradually increase the intensity and duration of the exercises over time.

3. Exercise preferences: Seniors should choose exercises that they enjoy and are more likely to stick with long-term. This may include chair exercises, yoga, water aerobics, or other low-impact exercises.

4. Exercise equipment: Seniors should also consider the equipment they will need for their chosen exercises. This may include resistance bands, weights, or other equipment that is appropriate for their fitness level and exercise program.

5. Safety precautions: Seniors should take appropriate safety precautions when exercising, including wearing appropriate clothing and footwear, staying hydrated, and warming up and cooling down properly.

By considering these factors before starting an exercise program, seniors can ensure that they are exercising safely and effectively for their individual needs and abilities. With regular exercise, seniors can improve their overall health and well-being, and enjoy a more active and fulfilling lifestyle.

2.3. How to Get Started with an Exercise Program

Starting an exercise program can be daunting, especially for seniors who may have physical limitations or health concerns. However, regular exercise is crucial for maintaining physical and mental health, and can even help prevent chronic diseases such as heart disease, diabetes, and osteoporosis.

Before starting any exercise program, it is important to consult with a healthcare provider to ensure that it is safe and appropriate for your individual needs and abilities. Once you have received the green light, it's time to get started!

First, choose an exercise or activity that you enjoy and that is appropriate for your fitness level. If you are new to exercise or have physical limitations, consider starting with chair exercises, balance exercises, or low-impact cardio exercises such as walking or cycling. If you are looking to build strength, consider incorporating strength training exercises using resistance bands or light weights.

It is important to start slowly and gradually increase the duration and intensity of your workouts as your fitness level improves. Aim for at least 30 minutes of moderate-intensity exercise most days of the week, or 150 minutes per week.

Stretching exercises are also important for maintaining flexibility and preventing injury. Incorporate stretching exercises into your workout routine, or consider attending a yoga class specifically designed for seniors. Water aerobics classes are another great option for low-impact cardio and strength training exercises.

Remember to listen to your body and rest when needed. If you experience pain or discomfort during exercise, stop and consult with your healthcare provider.

Starting an exercise program can be a challenge, but with the right mindset and approach, it can become a fun and rewarding part of your daily routine. Stick with it and enjoy the benefits of improved physical and mental health!

2.4. Common Exercise Mistakes to Avoid

Exercising is an essential aspect of maintaining a healthy lifestyle, regardless of age. As we age, our bodies undergo various changes that can make exercise challenging, but not impossible. However, as seniors, it's important to avoid common exercise mistakes that can lead to injuries, setbacks, or even discourage us from continuing with our fitness journey. Here are some common exercise mistakes to avoid when engaging in exercises for seniors:

1. Skipping Warm-up and Cool-down: Warm-up and cool-down exercises are crucial in preparing your body for physical activity and reducing the risk of injury. Skipping these exercises can cause your muscles to tighten, leading to muscle strain or injury.

2. Overdoing It: As seniors, we may feel the need to push ourselves harder to achieve our fitness goals. However, it's essential to listen to our bodies and avoid overdoing it. Overexertion can lead to muscle fatigue, injury, or even exhaustion.

3. Incorrect Form: Incorrect form during exercises can lead to injury or ineffective workouts. Ensure that you learn the proper form for each exercise and maintain it throughout the workout.

4. Holding Your Breath: Holding your breath during exercises can cause a spike in blood pressure and lead to dizziness or fainting. Remember to breathe evenly throughout the workout.

5. Neglecting Rest Days: Rest days are essential for muscle recovery and preventing burnout. Avoid overworking your muscles, and take a break when necessary.

6. Not Drinking Enough Water: Staying hydrated is crucial during exercise, especially for seniors. Drinking enough water helps maintain body temperature, lubricate joints, and prevent dehydration.

7. Ignoring Pain: Pain is your body's way of telling you that something is wrong. Ignoring pain can lead to further injury or setbacks. If you experience pain during exercise, stop and consult with your doctor or physical therapist.

In conclusion, avoiding these common exercise mistakes can help you stay safe, healthy, and motivated in your fitness journey. Remember to listen to your body, take breaks when necessary, and seek professional guidance if needed. Stay active and enjoy the benefits of exercises for seniors!

3. Chair Exercises for Seniors

3.1. Benefits of Chair Exercises

As we age, it's important to maintain our physical health and fitness. Regular exercise can help us stay healthy and active, but it can be challenging for seniors who may have mobility or balance issues. That's where chair exercises come in – they offer a convenient and safe way to stay active and improve overall health.

Here are some of the benefits of chair exercises for seniors:

1. Improved balance: Chair exercises can help improve balance and stability, which is important for preventing falls and injuries. Many chair exercises focus on core strength and stability, which can help improve balance and reduce the risk of falls.

2. Increased strength: Chair exercises can help seniors build strength and muscle mass, which can improve overall health and reduce the risk of injury. Many chair exercises focus on upper body strength, which is important for daily activities like carrying groceries or opening doors.

3. Low-impact cardio: Many chair exercises are designed to get the heart rate up and provide a cardiovascular workout, without putting stress on the joints. This is important for seniors who may have arthritis or other joint issues, and can help improve overall cardiovascular health.

4. Improved flexibility: Chair exercises can help improve flexibility and range of motion, which can reduce the risk of injury and improve daily activities. Many chair exercises focus on stretching and range of motion, which can help improve flexibility and reduce stiffness.

5. Convenience: Chair exercises can be done anywhere, anytime, making them a convenient way to stay active and healthy. Whether you're at home, at work, or traveling, you can always find a chair to use for exercise.

Overall, chair exercises are a great way for seniors to stay active and improve overall health and fitness. Whether you're looking to improve balance, strength, cardio, flexibility, or just stay active, chair exercises can help you achieve your goals in a safe and convenient way.

3.2. Chair Exercises for the Upper Body

As we age, our bodies undergo a number of changes that can impact our range of motion, muscle strength, and overall mobility. This can make it more difficult to engage in physical activity and can lead to a sedentary lifestyle. However, staying active is crucial for maintaining our health and wellbeing as we age.

Fortunately, there are a number of exercises that can be done while seated in a chair that can help improve upper body strength and mobility. These exercises are low-impact and can be modified to meet a range of physical abilities.

One simple chair exercise for the upper body is the seated arm raise. To do this exercise, sit upright in a chair with your feet flat on the ground. Hold a light weight in each hand (or use water bottles or cans of soup if you don't have weights) and raise your arms out to your sides, bringing them up to shoulder height. Hold for a few seconds and then slowly lower your arms back down to your sides. Repeat for several repetitions.

Another great exercise for the upper body is the seated row. Sit on the edge of your chair with your feet flat on the ground. Hold a resistance band in front of you with both hands, palms facing each other. Pull the band towards your chest, squeezing your shoulder blades together. Slowly release the band back to the starting position and repeat for several repetitions.

If you have access to a set of hand weights, you can also do bicep curls and tricep extensions while seated in a chair. To do bicep curls, hold a weight in each hand and curl your arms up towards your shoulders. To do tricep extensions, hold a weight in one hand and lift it up behind your head, bending your arm at the elbow.

Incorporating chair exercises for the upper body into your daily routine can help improve your strength and mobility, making it easier to stay active and engaged in the activities you love. Remember to always consult with your healthcare provider before starting any new exercise program, and to modify exercises as needed to meet your individual needs and abilities.

3.3. Chair Exercises for the Lower Body

As we age, it's important to maintain our physical health and fitness. However, some seniors may struggle with traditional exercises due to mobility or balance issues.

Chair exercises for the lower body are a great way to stay active and healthy without putting too much strain on the body. These exercises can be done from the comfort of a chair and are perfect for seniors who are looking to improve their leg strength and flexibility.

1. Leg lifts: Sit on a chair with your feet flat on the ground. Lift one leg straight out in front of you and hold for a few seconds before lowering it back down. Repeat on the other leg.

2. Knee extensions: Sit on a chair with your feet flat on the ground. Lift one knee up towards your chest and hold for a few seconds before lowering it back down. Repeat on the other leg.

3. Calf raises: Sit on a chair with your feet flat on the ground. Lift your heels off the ground and hold for a few seconds before lowering them back down.

4. Seated squats: Sit on a chair with your feet flat on the ground. Slowly stand up from the chair and then sit back down. Repeat for a few reps.

These chair exercises for the lower body can be done daily or as often as needed. They are a great way to improve leg strength and flexibility without putting too much strain on the body. It's important to remember to start slowly and gradually increase the intensity of the exercises as you become more comfortable and confident.

In addition to chair exercises, seniors can also incorporate balance exercises, strength training exercises, low-impact cardio exercises, stretching exercises, water aerobics

exercises, and yoga exercises into their fitness routine.
These exercises can help improve overall physical health
and fitness and keep seniors active and healthy for years to
come.

3.4. Chair Exercises for Flexibility and Balance

As we age, it's important to maintain flexibility and balance
to prevent falls and maintain independence. Chair exercises
are a great way to improve both flexibility and balance
while providing a safe and stable environment.

Here are some chair exercises you can try:

1. Sit-to-stand: Sit on the edge of the chair with your feet
flat on the ground. Using your leg muscles, stand up and
then slowly sit back down. Repeat 10-15 times.

2. Leg lifts: Sit on the edge of the chair with your back
straight and hands resting on your thighs. Lift one leg
straight out in front of you, hold for a few seconds, then
lower it back down. Repeat on the other leg. Do 10-15 reps
on each leg.

3. Seated twists: Sit on the chair with your feet flat on the
ground. Twist your upper body to the right, holding onto
the back of the chair with your left hand. Hold for a few
seconds, then twist to the left, holding onto the back of the
chair with your right hand. Repeat 10-15 times on each
side.

4. Arm circles: Sit on the chair with your back straight and
feet flat on the ground. Raise your arms out to the sides and

make small circles with your hands. Gradually increase the size of the circles. Do 10-15 reps in each direction.

5. Knee lifts: Sit tall in the chair with your feet flat on the ground. Lift your right knee towards your chest, then lower it back down. Repeat on the left side. Do 10-15 reps on each side.

Remember to breathe deeply and stay focused on your movements. These exercises can be done daily or as part of a regular exercise routine. By incorporating chair exercises into your daily routine, you can improve your flexibility and balance, leading to a healthier and more active lifestyle.

4. Balance Exercises for Seniors

4.1. The Importance of Balance Exercises for Seniors

As we age, our bodies undergo various changes that affect our balance. We may experience a decrease in muscle mass, changes in vision, and a decrease in flexibility, all of which can lead to an increased risk of falls. However, by incorporating balance exercises into our daily routine, we can improve our stability and reduce the risk of falls.

Balance exercises are crucial for seniors because they help improve proprioception, which is the body's ability to sense its position in space. These exercises also help strengthen the muscles in the lower body, which are essential for maintaining balance.

One of the best ways to incorporate balance exercises into your daily routine is through chair exercises. These exercises are low-impact, which means they do not put too much pressure on your joints, making them ideal for seniors who may have arthritis or other joint-related conditions.

Another excellent way to improve your balance is through strength training exercises. These exercises help build the muscles in your legs, hips, and core, which are essential for maintaining balance. Some examples of strength training exercises include squats, lunges, and leg lifts.

Low-impact cardio exercises are also great for improving your balance. These exercises include walking, cycling, and swimming, all of which can help improve your cardiovascular health and strengthen your lower body muscles.

Stretching exercises are also essential for seniors, as they help improve flexibility and range of motion. By incorporating stretching into your daily routine, you can improve your balance and reduce the risk of falls.

Water aerobics exercises are an excellent option for seniors who may have joint-related conditions. These exercises are low-impact and can help improve cardiovascular health, strengthen the muscles, and improve balance.

Finally, yoga exercises are another great option for seniors. Yoga helps improve flexibility, strength, and balance, making it an ideal exercise for seniors.

In conclusion, incorporating balance exercises into your daily routine is crucial for seniors. By improving your stability and reducing the risk of falls, you can enjoy a healthier and more active lifestyle. Whether it's through chair exercises, strength training, low-impact cardio, stretching, water aerobics, or yoga, there are plenty of options available to help you improve your balance and maintain your overall health and well-being.

4.2. Balance Exercises for the Lower Body

Balance exercises for the lower body are essential for seniors because they help prevent falls and maintain independence. As we age, our balance can be affected due to changes in the inner ear, vision, and muscle strength.

Fortunately, there are several exercises that seniors can do to improve their balance and stability.

One of the simplest balance exercises for seniors is standing on one leg. Stand near a wall or chair for support and lift one leg off the ground. Hold for 10-15 seconds and then switch legs. Repeat 5-10 times on each leg. This exercise can be progressed by closing your eyes or standing on a pillow or cushion.

Another great balance exercise is heel-to-toe walking. Place one foot directly in front of the other, so that the heel of the front foot touches the toes of the back foot. Walk heel-to-toe in a straight line for 10-15 steps and then turn around and walk back. Repeat 5-10 times.

Seniors can also benefit from practicing the yoga pose Warrior III. Stand with your feet hip-width apart and arms at your sides. Bend forward and lift one leg behind you, keeping your arms and torso parallel to the floor. Hold for 10-15 seconds and then switch legs. Repeat 5-10 times on each leg.

Finally, seniors can try the exercise known as the chair squat. Stand in front of a chair with your feet shoulder-width apart. Slowly lower yourself down to sit in the chair, but don't actually sit down. Instead, hover just above the chair for a few seconds before standing back up. Repeat 10-15 times.

In conclusion, balance exercises for the lower body are crucial for seniors to maintain their independence and prevent falls. Incorporating these exercises into your daily routine can improve your balance and stability, allowing you to live an active and healthy lifestyle. Remember to start slowly and progress gradually, and always check with your doctor before beginning any new exercise program.

4.3. Balance Exercises for the Upper Body

As we age, maintaining balance becomes increasingly important. Falls are one of the leading causes of injury among seniors, and improving balance can go a long way in preventing them. While most balance exercises focus on the lower body, it's important not to neglect the upper body. Strengthening the muscles in your shoulders, arms, and core can improve overall stability and make it easier to maintain balance.

Here are some simple balance exercises that focus on the upper body:

1. Wall Push-Ups - Stand facing a wall with your feet shoulder-width apart. Place your hands on the wall at shoulder height. Slowly lower your chest towards the wall, keeping your elbows close to your body. Push back up to the starting position. Repeat for 10-15 reps.

2. Shoulder Circles - Stand with your feet shoulder-width apart and your arms at your sides. Slowly raise your arms out to the sides, keeping them straight. Make small circles with your arms, first going forward and then backward. Repeat for 10-15 reps in each direction.

3. Arm Raises - Stand with your feet shoulder-width apart and your arms at your sides. Slowly raise your arms out in front of you, keeping them straight. Raise them as high as you can, then slowly lower them back down. Repeat for 10-15 reps.

4. Seated Shoulder Shrugs - Sit in a chair with your feet flat on the floor. Lift your shoulders up towards your ears, then release them back down. Repeat for 10-15 reps.

5. Arm Circles - Sit in a chair with your feet flat on the floor. Extend your arms out to the sides, keeping them at shoulder height. Make small circles with your arms, first going forward and then backward. Repeat for 10-15 reps in each direction.

Remember to breathe deeply and maintain good posture throughout these exercises. As you get stronger, you can increase the number of reps or add light weights for extra resistance. By incorporating these simple upper body balance exercises into your routine, you can improve your overall stability and reduce your risk of falls.

4.4. Balance Exercises for Overall Balance and Stability

Balance is an essential aspect of daily life, especially as we age. It helps us to maintain stability, prevent falls and injuries, and perform daily activities with ease. Balance exercises are an effective way to improve balance and stability, and they are suitable for seniors of all fitness levels.

Here are some effective balance exercises that will help you improve your balance, stability, and coordination:

1. Single-leg stance: Stand on one leg and hold the position for 30 seconds. Repeat on the other leg.

2. Heel-to-toe walk: Walk in a straight line, placing one foot in front of the other, heel to toe.

3. Leg swings: Stand behind a chair and swing one leg forward and backward, then side to side.

4. Side leg raises: Stand behind a chair and lift one leg out to the side, then lower it back down. Repeat on the other leg.

5. Wall push-ups: Stand facing a wall and place your hands on the wall. Lean forward, bending your elbows, and then push yourself back up.

6. Balance ball exercises: Use a balance ball to perform exercises such as sitting on the ball and lifting one leg, or standing on the ball and rolling it back and forth.

7. Yoga poses: Yoga is an excellent way to improve balance and stability. Poses such as tree pose, warrior pose, and half-moon pose are particularly beneficial.

Balance exercises can be performed throughout the day, and you can start with just a few minutes of exercise per day and gradually increase the duration and intensity. Additionally, incorporating balance exercises into your daily routine can be a fun and effective way to improve your overall fitness and well-being.

In conclusion, balance exercises are essential for seniors to maintain overall balance and stability. Whether you are a beginner or an experienced fitness enthusiast, incorporating these exercises into your routine will help you improve your balance, coordination, and prevent falls and injuries. Remember to always consult with your healthcare provider before starting any new exercise program.

5. Strength Training Exercises for Seniors

5.1. Benefits of Strength Training for Seniors

Strength training is an essential aspect of exercise for seniors. As we age, our muscles tend to weaken, which can lead to a range of mobility problems. However, strength training can help to combat this decline and improve overall physical functioning. In this chapter, we will discuss the benefits of strength training for seniors and why it should be a crucial part of any exercise routine.

One of the most significant benefits of strength training for seniors is the increase in muscle mass and strength. As we age, we tend to lose muscle mass, which can lead to a variety of health problems. However, strength training can help to improve muscle mass and strength, which can lead to better balance, coordination, and mobility. This, in turn, can help to prevent falls and other injuries.

Strength training can also help to improve bone density. As we age, our bones tend to become weaker, which can lead to osteoporosis and other bone-related conditions. However, strength training can help to increase bone density, which can help to prevent these conditions from occurring.

Strength training can also help to improve flexibility. As we age, our joints tend to become stiffer, which can lead to mobility problems. However, strength training can help to increase flexibility, which can help to improve range of motion and reduce the risk of injury.

Another significant benefit of strength training for seniors is the improvement in overall health. Strength training can help to lower blood pressure, reduce the risk of diabetes, improve cholesterol levels, and boost the immune system. This can lead to better overall health and a reduced risk of chronic diseases.

In conclusion, strength training is an essential aspect of exercise for seniors. It can help to improve muscle mass and strength, increase bone density, improve flexibility, and improve overall health. Therefore, seniors should incorporate strength training into their exercise routine to maintain good health and well-being.

5.2. Strength Training Exercises for the Upper Body

Strength training exercises for the upper body are crucial for seniors who want to maintain their independence and functional abilities. As we age, our muscles naturally weaken, making it more difficult to perform everyday tasks such as carrying groceries or reaching for objects on high shelves. However, regular strength training exercises can help to slow down this process and keep our upper body muscles strong and functional.

One of the most effective upper body strength training exercises for seniors is the chest press. This exercise targets the muscles in the chest, shoulders, and triceps, and can be performed using dumbbells or resistance bands. To perform the chest press, sit on a chair with your feet flat on the ground and a dumbbell or resistance band in each hand.

Bring your arms up to shoulder height, with your elbows bent at a 90-degree angle. Then, push the weights or bands forward, straightening your arms out in front of you. Repeat for 10-15 repetitions.

Another effective upper body strength training exercise for seniors is the shoulder press. This exercise targets the muscles in the shoulders and upper back, and can also be performed using dumbbells or resistance bands. To perform the shoulder press, sit on a chair with your feet flat on the ground and a dumbbell or resistance band in each hand. Bring your arms up to shoulder height, with your elbows bent at a 90-degree angle. Then, push the weights or bands up overhead, straightening your arms fully. Repeat for 10-15 repetitions.

In addition to the chest press and shoulder press, seniors can also benefit from exercises that target the biceps, triceps, and upper back muscles. Bicep curls, tricep extensions, and rows are all effective exercises that can be performed using dumbbells or resistance bands.

Overall, incorporating upper body strength training exercises into your exercise routine can help you maintain your functional abilities and independence as you age. Always be sure to consult with a healthcare professional before starting any new exercise program, and start with light weights or resistance bands if you are new to strength training.

5.3. Strength Training Exercises for the Lower Body

Strength training is an essential part of active aging. Building muscle mass and strength helps to improve balance, mobility, and protect against falls. The lower body is particularly important to focus on as it is responsible for our ability to stand, walk, and climb stairs.

Here are some strength training exercises for the lower body that are suitable for seniors:

1. Squats

Squats are an excellent exercise for strengthening the muscles in your legs, hips, and glutes. You can start with chair squats by using a sturdy chair as a prop. Stand in front of the chair with your feet shoulder-width apart, then lower your body down towards the chair as if you were going to sit down. Once your hips touch the chair, stand back up. Repeat for 10-15 repetitions.

2. Lunges

Lunges are another great exercise for strengthening the legs, hips, and glutes. Stand with your feet hip-width apart, then step forward with one foot and lower your body down towards the ground. Make sure your front knee does not go past your toes. Push back up with your front foot and return to the starting position. Repeat on the other side. Aim for 10-15 repetitions on each leg.

3. Calf Raises

Calf raises are an excellent exercise for strengthening the muscles in your calves. Stand with your feet hip-width apart, then raise your heels off the ground as high as you

can go. Hold for a few seconds, then lower back down.
Aim for 10-15 repetitions.

4. Bridges

Bridges are an excellent exercise for strengthening the
glutes and lower back muscles. Lie on your back with your
knees bent and your feet flat on the ground. Lift your hips
up towards the ceiling, squeezing your glutes at the top.
Lower back down to the starting position. Aim for 10-15
repetitions.

As with any exercise program, it is essential to start slowly
and gradually increase your intensity. Always listen to your
body and stop if you experience any pain or discomfort.
Incorporating strength training exercises for the lower body
into your routine can help you maintain your mobility,
balance, and independence as you age.

5.4. How to Progress with Strength Training Exercises

Strength training exercises are a crucial part of any fitness
routine, regardless of age. For seniors, it's important to
focus on exercises that build and maintain muscle mass, as
well as improve bone density and overall strength. Here are
some tips on how to progress with your strength training
exercises:

1. Start with light weights or resistance bands: If you're
new to strength training, it's important to start with lighter
weights or resistance bands to avoid injury. Focus on using

proper form and technique to build a foundation for more challenging exercises.

2. Increase weight gradually: As you become more comfortable with your exercises, gradually increase the weight or resistance to continue challenging yourself. Remember to always listen to your body and avoid pushing yourself too hard.

3. Incorporate compound exercises: Compound exercises work multiple muscle groups at once, making them more efficient and effective. Examples include squats, lunges, and push-ups.

4. Don't forget about rest and recovery: Strength training can be taxing on the body, so it's important to allow for proper rest and recovery time. Aim for at least one day of rest between strength training sessions and incorporate stretching or low-impact cardio exercises on your off days.

5. Seek guidance from a professional: If you're unsure about proper form or which exercises to incorporate into your routine, consider working with a certified personal trainer or physical therapist. They can help develop a personalized plan that fits your individual needs and goals.

Remember, strength training is just one component of a well-rounded fitness routine. Be sure to also incorporate balance, cardio, stretching, and other exercises to achieve optimal health and wellness.

6. Low-Impact Cardio Exercises for Seniors

6.1. Benefits of Low-impact Cardio Exercises

Low-impact cardio exercises are exercises that are gentle on the joints and are suitable for seniors who may have arthritis, osteoporosis, or other conditions that limit their range of motion. These exercises are an excellent way to get the heart rate up, burn calories, and improve cardiovascular health without putting too much strain on the body. Here are some of the benefits that seniors can enjoy from low-impact cardio exercises:

1. Improves heart health

Low-impact cardio exercises can help improve heart health by strengthening the heart muscle and improving blood circulation. Studies have shown that low-impact cardio exercises such as walking, cycling, and swimming can lower blood pressure, reduce the risk of heart disease, and improve overall cardiovascular health.

2. Helps with weight management

Low-impact cardio exercises are an effective way to burn calories and maintain a healthy weight. These exercises can help seniors to reduce body fat, increase muscle mass, and improve metabolism. This can help to prevent obesity and reduce the risk of chronic diseases such as diabetes, high blood pressure, and heart disease.

3. Builds endurance and stamina

Low-impact cardio exercises can help seniors to build endurance and stamina, making it easier for them to perform daily activities such as walking, climbing stairs, and carrying groceries. These exercises can also help to improve balance and coordination, reducing the risk of falls and injuries.

4. Reduces stress and anxiety

Low-impact cardio exercises can help to reduce stress and anxiety by releasing endorphins, which are natural mood-enhancing chemicals in the brain. These exercises can also help seniors to feel more relaxed and improve their overall sense of well-being.

5. Promotes better sleep

Low-impact cardio exercises can help to promote better sleep by reducing stress, improving mood, and increasing relaxation. Seniors who engage in regular low-impact cardio exercises may find that they are able to fall asleep more easily and sleep more soundly throughout the night.

In conclusion, low-impact cardio exercises are an excellent way for seniors to improve their overall health and well-being. These exercises can help to improve heart health, manage weight, build endurance and stamina, reduce stress and anxiety, and promote better sleep. Seniors who are looking for a gentle and effective way to stay active should consider incorporating low-impact cardio exercises into their exercise routine.

6.2. Low-impact Cardio Exercises for the Upper Body

As we age, it's important to maintain a healthy and active lifestyle. One way to do this is through low-impact cardio exercises that focus on the upper body. These exercises are gentle on the joints and can help improve cardiovascular health, muscle strength, and overall fitness.

Here are some low-impact cardio exercises for the upper body that seniors can try:

1. Arm circles - Stand with your feet shoulder-width apart and extend your arms out to the side. Make small circles with your arms, gradually increasing the size of the circles. Reverse the direction of the circles after a few repetitions.

2. Seated rowing - Sit on a chair with your feet flat on the ground and a resistance band looped around your feet. Hold the ends of the band with your hands and pull your elbows back, squeezing your shoulder blades together. Release slowly and repeat.

3. Wall push-ups - Stand facing a wall with your feet about shoulder-width apart. Place your hands on the wall at shoulder height and slowly lower your chest towards the wall. Push back up to the starting position and repeat.

4. Shoulder rolls - Sit on a chair with your feet flat on the ground and your back straight. Roll your shoulders forward, up, back, and down in a circular motion. Repeat in the opposite direction.

5. Arm raises - Stand with your feet shoulder-width apart and your arms at your sides. Lift your arms out to the side and up towards your shoulders, then lower them back down to your sides. Repeat.

Remember to start slowly and gradually increase the intensity and duration of your workouts. It's also important to listen to your body and stop if you feel any pain or discomfort. These low-impact cardio exercises can be done at home or in a group fitness class, making them a convenient and effective way for seniors to stay active and healthy.

6.3. Low-impact Cardio Exercises for the Lower Body

Low-impact cardio exercises are great for seniors who want to improve their cardiovascular health and endurance without putting stress on their joints. These exercises can be done in the comfort of your own home or at a gym. Here are some low-impact cardio exercises for the lower body:

1. Walking – Walking is a great low-impact exercise that can be done almost anywhere. You can walk outdoors or indoors on a treadmill. Start with a 10-minute walk and gradually increase the duration as you get stronger.

2. Cycling – Cycling is a great low-impact exercise that can be done on a stationary bike or outdoors on a regular bike. This exercise is great for building endurance and improving cardiovascular health.

3. Swimming – Swimming is a great low-impact exercise that is easy on the joints. It is a great exercise for seniors who have arthritis or other joint problems. Swimming can also help improve your flexibility and range of motion.

4. Elliptical – The elliptical is a low-impact exercise machine that is great for seniors. It can help improve your cardiovascular health and endurance without putting stress on your joints.

5. Dancing – Dancing is a fun way to get your heart rate up and improve your cardiovascular health. You can dance at home or take a dance class at your local gym.

6. Step aerobics – Step aerobics is a low-impact exercise that can be done at home or in a group fitness class. This exercise is great for improving your cardiovascular health and endurance.

Remember to start slowly and gradually increase the intensity and duration of your workouts. Always listen to your body and stop if you experience any pain or discomfort. Low-impact cardio exercises are a great way to improve your cardiovascular health and endurance without putting stress on your joints. Incorporate these exercises into your workout routine to stay active and healthy.

6.4. How to Progress with Low-impact Cardio Exercises

As we age, it is important to keep our bodies active and moving, but it can be challenging to find exercises that are low-impact and gentle on our joints. Fortunately, there are many options for low-impact cardio exercises that can help improve cardiovascular health, strengthen muscles, and increase endurance without putting stress on the body.

One of the best low-impact cardio exercises for seniors is walking. Walking is a great way to get your heart rate up and burn calories, and it can be done indoors or outdoors, depending on your preference. If you have access to a treadmill, you can adjust the incline and speed to increase the intensity of your workout.

Another great low-impact cardio exercise is cycling. Cycling can be done on a stationary bike or outdoors, and it is a great way to work your leg muscles while improving cardiovascular health. You can adjust the resistance and speed to challenge yourself and increase your endurance over time.

Swimming and water aerobics are also excellent low-impact cardio exercises for seniors. Water provides resistance, which can help build strength and endurance while reducing stress on the joints. Swimming and water aerobics are also great options for those with arthritis or other joint problems.

Dancing is another fun and effective low-impact cardio exercise for seniors. You can dance to your favorite music at home or join a dance class for a social and enjoyable workout. Dancing can improve balance, coordination, and flexibility while getting your heart rate up.

It is important to start slowly and gradually increase the intensity and duration of your workouts over time. It is also important to listen to your body and rest when needed. Remember to stay hydrated and wear comfortable, supportive shoes and clothing.

Incorporating low-impact cardio exercises into your fitness routine can help improve your overall health and well-being. Whether you prefer walking, cycling, swimming, dancing, or another form of low-impact cardio, finding an exercise that you enjoy can make all the difference in staying active and healthy as you age.

7. Stretching Exercises for Seniors

7.1. Benefits of Stretching for Seniors

Stretching is a crucial component of physical fitness, regardless of age. However, it becomes even more important for seniors to incorporate stretching exercises into their daily routine. The benefits of stretching for seniors are numerous and include increased flexibility, improved range of motion, reduced risk of injury, and enhanced overall well-being.

One of the primary benefits of stretching for seniors is increased flexibility. As we age, our muscles and joints become stiffer, making it more challenging to move freely. However, stretching can help improve flexibility, making it easier to perform daily activities such as bending, reaching, and walking. Stretching can also help improve balance and coordination, which can reduce the risk of falls in seniors.

Improved range of motion is another significant benefit of stretching for seniors. By regularly stretching, seniors can improve their joint mobility, making it easier to move their limbs and perform activities that require a greater range of motion. This increased range of motion can also help reduce joint pain and stiffness, which is a common problem for many seniors.

Stretching can also help reduce the risk of injury in seniors. By improving flexibility and range of motion, seniors are less likely to experience strains, sprains, or other injuries that can result from sudden movements or accidents.

Stretching can also help improve circulation, which can reduce the risk of blood clots, heart disease, and other health conditions.

Finally, stretching can enhance overall wellbeing in seniors. Stretching can help reduce stress and tension, promote relaxation, and improve mood. Regular stretching can also help improve sleep quality, which is essential for overall health and wellbeing.

In conclusion, stretching is an essential component of physical fitness for seniors. It can help increase flexibility, improve range of motion, reduce the risk of injury, and enhance overall wellbeing. Seniors should incorporate stretching exercises into their daily routine to enjoy these benefits and maintain optimal physical and mental health.

7.2. Stretching Exercises for the Upper Body

Stretching exercises for the upper body are a great way for seniors to improve their range of motion, flexibility, and posture. These exercises can be done at home or in a group setting and require little to no equipment.

One of the most common stretching exercises for the upper body is the shoulder stretch. To perform this exercise, stand with your feet shoulder-width apart and your arms at your sides. Slowly raise your right arm and bring it across your body, holding it with your left hand for 10-15 seconds. Repeat on the other side.

Another effective upper body stretching exercise is the triceps stretch. To do this, stand with your feet shoulder-width apart and raise your right arm above your head. Bend your right elbow and reach your right hand behind your head, holding your elbow with your left hand for 10-15 seconds. Repeat on the other side.

The chest stretch is also a great upper body stretching exercise. To perform this exercise, stand facing a wall with your arms outstretched and your palms against the wall. Slowly lean forward, feeling the stretch in your chest and shoulders. Hold for 10-15 seconds.

In addition to these stretches, seniors can also benefit from incorporating yoga into their exercise routine. Yoga focuses on stretching and strengthening the entire body, including the upper body. Poses such as downward dog, upward dog, and the warrior series can help improve posture, increase flexibility, and reduce stiffness in the upper body.

Overall, stretching exercises for the upper body are an important part of any senior's exercise routine. These exercises can help improve flexibility, range of motion, and posture, leading to a better quality of life. Seniors should consult with a healthcare provider before beginning any new exercise program.

7.3. Stretching Exercises for the Lower Body

Stretching exercises are an essential part of any fitness routine, especially for seniors who want to maintain their flexibility and prevent injuries. In this section, we will cover some simple and effective stretching exercises for the lower body that seniors can easily do at home.

1. Seated Forward Bend: Sit on a chair with your feet flat on the ground. Slowly bend forward at the hips and reach towards your toes. Hold for 10-15 seconds and slowly come back up. This stretch helps to stretch your hamstrings and lower back.

2. Quad Stretch: Stand behind a chair and hold onto the backrest for support. Bend your right knee and bring your heel towards your buttocks. Hold for 10-15 seconds and repeat on the other side. This stretch helps to stretch your quadriceps.

3. Hip Flexor Stretch: Stand facing a chair and place your left foot on the seat of the chair. Keep your right foot on the ground and slowly lean forward until you feel a stretch in your left hip. Hold for 10-15 seconds and repeat on the other side. This stretch helps to stretch your hip flexors.

4. Calf Stretch: Stand facing a wall with your hands on the wall for support. Step your right foot back and keep your heel on the ground. Lean forward until you feel a stretch in your right calf. Hold for 10-15 seconds and repeat on the other side.

5. Ankle Circles: Sit on a chair with your feet flat on the ground. Slowly rotate your feet in a circular motion, first clockwise and then counterclockwise. This stretch helps to improve ankle mobility.

Remember to breathe deeply and hold each stretch for 10-15 seconds. Don't force your body into any uncomfortable positions and stop if you feel any pain. Incorporating these stretching exercises into your daily routine can help you maintain your flexibility and mobility as you age.

7.4. How to Progress with Stretching Exercises

Stretching exercises are an essential component of any fitness routine, especially for seniors. As we age, our muscles and joints become less flexible, making it harder to move and perform daily activities. Regular stretching exercises can help improve flexibility, reduce the risk of injury, and enhance overall physical performance.

Here are some tips on how to progress with stretching exercises:

1. Start slowly

If you are new to stretching exercises, it is important to start slowly and gradually increase the intensity and duration of your stretches. Begin with simple stretches that target the major muscle groups, such as the hamstrings, quadriceps, and back muscles. Hold each stretch for 10-30 seconds and repeat 2-3 times.

2. Focus on breathing

Breathing is an important aspect of any stretching exercise. Inhale deeply before each stretch and exhale slowly as you move into the stretch. This will help you relax and increase the effectiveness of the stretch.

3. Use props

Using props such as blocks, straps, and bolsters can help you achieve deeper stretches and enhance your overall flexibility. For example, if you have tight hamstrings, you can use a strap to help you reach your toes during a seated forward fold.

4. Don't overdo it

While stretching is essential for maintaining flexibility, it is important not to overdo it. Stretching too much or too often can lead to muscle strains, joint pain, and other injuries. Listen to your body and stop if you experience any pain or discomfort.

5. Incorporate variety

To keep your stretching routine interesting and effective, it is important to incorporate a variety of exercises. Try different types of stretches, such as static, dynamic, and PNF (proprioceptive neuromuscular facilitation) stretches, to target different muscles and enhance your overall flexibility.

In conclusion, stretching exercises are an essential component of any fitness routine, especially for seniors. By starting slowly, focusing on breathing, using props, not overdoing it, and incorporating variety, you can progress with stretching exercises and improve your overall physical performance.

8. Water Aerobics Exercises for Seniors

8.1. Benefits of Water Aerobics for Seniors

Water aerobics is a low-impact exercise that can provide a range of benefits for seniors. This type of exercise involves performing aerobic exercises in a pool, where the buoyancy of the water helps reduce the impact on the joints and muscles. Water aerobics is a great way for seniors to stay active and healthy, and can provide the following benefits:

1. Low-impact exercise: As mentioned, water aerobics is a low-impact exercise that can be gentler on the joints and muscles than other forms of exercise. This makes it an ideal exercise for seniors who may have arthritis or other joint issues.

2. Improves cardiovascular health: Water aerobics is a great form of cardio exercise, which can help improve heart health and circulation. This type of exercise can also help lower blood pressure and reduce the risk of heart disease.

3. Builds strength and endurance: Water aerobics can help build strength and endurance, which can improve overall fitness and quality of life. This type of exercise can also help seniors maintain independence and perform daily activities more easily.

4. Improves balance and coordination: The resistance of the water can help improve balance and coordination, which can reduce the risk of falls and other accidents.

5. Provides a social outlet: Water aerobics classes can be a great way for seniors to meet new people and socialize. This can provide a sense of community and support, which can be important for overall health and well-being.

Overall, water aerobics is a great exercise option for seniors. It is low-impact, improves cardiovascular health, builds strength and endurance, improves balance and coordination, and provides a social outlet. Seniors who are interested in trying water aerobics should consult with their doctor first, and look for classes specifically designed for seniors.

8.2. Water Aerobics Exercises for the Upper Body

Water aerobics is a low-impact exercise that is perfect for seniors who want to improve their upper body strength. The resistance of the water provides a natural and gentle workout, which is ideal for those with joint pain or mobility issues. Here are some water aerobics exercises that can help you build upper body strength:

1. Water walking: This exercise is perfect for seniors who want to improve their overall body strength. Simply walk back and forth in the shallow end of the pool, lifting your knees and swinging your arms as you go. This exercise will work your core, arms, and legs.

2. Arm curls: Using water weights or dumbbells, stand in chest-deep water and extend your arms out to the sides. Slowly bring them back in, lifting the weights as you go. This exercise will work your biceps and shoulders.

3. Push-ups: Stand in waist-deep water and position yourself against the pool edge. Push your body up and down, using the edge as a support. This exercise will work your chest, shoulders, and triceps.

4. Arm circles: Stand in chest-deep water and extend your arms out to the sides. Slowly make big circles with your arms. This exercise will work your shoulders and upper back.

5. Water punches: Stand in waist-deep water and punch the water, alternating arms. This exercise will work your arms and shoulders.

6. Flutter kicks: Hold onto the pool edge and kick your legs back and forth. This exercise will work your abs, legs, and glutes.

7. Pool noodle curls: Hold a pool noodle in front of you and curl it up to your chest. This exercise will work your biceps and shoulders.

Water aerobics is a fun and effective way to improve your upper body strength. By incorporating these exercises into your routine, you can feel stronger and more confident in your daily activities. Remember to always consult with your doctor before starting any new exercise program.

8.3. Water Aerobics Exercises for the Lower Body

Water aerobics exercises are a great way for seniors to stay active and improve their overall health. These exercises not only help to increase strength and flexibility, but they also provide a low-impact workout that is gentle on joints.

When it comes to water aerobics exercises for the lower body, there are a variety of options to choose from. Here are some exercises to consider:

1. **Leg lifts**: Stand in waist-deep water with your feet together. Raise one leg out to the side and hold for a few seconds before lowering it back down. Repeat on the other side. This exercise targets the hip and outer thigh muscles.

2. **Knee lifts**: Stand in waist-deep water with your feet together. Lift one knee up towards your chest and hold for a few seconds before lowering it back down. Repeat on the other side. This exercise targets the quadriceps muscles.

3. **Water walking**: Walk forward and backward in waist-deep water. This exercise targets the lower body muscles, including the glutes, hamstrings, and calves.

4. **Squats**: Stand in shoulder-deep water with your feet shoulder-width apart. Lower down into a squat position and hold for a few seconds before standing back up. This exercise targets the quadriceps, glutes, and hamstrings.

5. **Water jogging**: Jog in place in waist-deep water. This exercise provides a low-impact cardio workout that targets the lower body muscles.

Remember to start slowly and gradually increase the intensity of your water aerobics exercises. It's also important to listen to your body and stop if you experience any pain or discomfort.

Incorporating water aerobics exercises into your workout routine is a great way to improve your overall health and stay active as you age. So, grab your swimsuit and hit the pool!

8.4. How to Progress with Water Aerobics Exercises

Water aerobics exercises are a great way for seniors to stay active and healthy. Not only is it a low-impact form of exercise, but it also provides resistance that can help build strength and improve cardiovascular health. Here are some tips on how to progress with water aerobics exercises:

1. Start with the basics: If you're new to water aerobics, start with the basics. This means doing simple movements like marching in place, leg lifts, and arm circles. Focus on getting used to the water and the resistance it provides.

2. Increase the intensity: Once you're comfortable with the basics, it's time to increase the intensity of your water aerobics exercises. You can do this by adding more resistance, such as using hand weights or resistance bands. You can also increase the speed of your movements to get your heart rate up.

3. Try new exercises: Don't be afraid to try new water aerobics exercises. There are many different movements you can do in the water, such as jumping jacks, bicycling, and water walking. Trying new exercises can help prevent boredom and keep your workouts challenging.

4. Challenge yourself: As you get stronger and more comfortable in the water, challenge yourself by increasing the duration of your workouts or trying more advanced movements. You can also try interval training by alternating between high-intensity and low-intensity exercises.

5. Work with a professional: If you're unsure about how to progress with your water aerobics exercises, consider working with a professional. A certified water aerobics instructor can help you create a customized workout plan and provide guidance on how to progress safely.

In conclusion, water aerobics exercises are a great way for seniors to stay active and healthy. By starting with the basics, increasing the intensity, trying new exercises, challenging yourself, and working with a professional, you can progress with your water aerobics workouts and continue to see improvements in your health and fitness.

9. Yoga Exercises for Seniors

9.1. Benefits of Yoga for Seniors

Yoga has been practiced for centuries and has become increasingly popular as a form of exercise for people of all ages, including seniors. The benefits of yoga for seniors are many and varied, and can help improve overall health and well-being.

One of the main benefits of yoga for seniors is improved flexibility. As we age, our joints become stiffer and less flexible, which can lead to a range of health issues. Yoga helps to improve flexibility by stretching and lengthening the muscles, which in turn helps to improve range of motion and reduce the risk of injury.

Yoga can also help to improve balance and stability, which is especially important for seniors. Many yoga poses require the practitioner to balance on one foot or maintain a steady posture, which can help to improve balance and reduce the risk of falls.

Another benefit of yoga for seniors is improved strength and muscle tone. Yoga poses require the practitioner to engage and activate various muscle groups, which can help to build strength and improve muscle tone. This can lead to improved overall fitness and reduced risk of injury.

Yoga is also a low-impact form of exercise, which makes it ideal for seniors who may have joint pain or other health issues that limit their ability to engage in high-impact activities. Many yoga poses can be modified to suit individual needs, making it a safe and accessible form of exercise for seniors of all fitness levels.

In addition to physical benefits, yoga can also help to improve mental health and well-being. The practice of yoga has been shown to reduce stress and anxiety, improve mood, and promote relaxation and mindfulness. This can be especially beneficial for seniors who may be dealing with issues such as depression or anxiety.

Overall, the benefits of yoga for seniors are many and varied, and can help to improve overall health and well-being. Whether practiced alone or as part of a larger exercise routine, yoga is a valuable tool for seniors looking to maintain their physical and mental health as they age.

9.2. Yoga Poses for Flexibility and Balance

Yoga is an ancient practice that has gained popularity in recent years due to its numerous health benefits. It is a low-impact form of exercise that is perfect for seniors who want to improve their flexibility and balance. In this section, we will discuss the best yoga poses for seniors who want to maintain their flexibility and balance as they age.

1. Tree pose (Vrikshasana)

The tree pose is a great way to improve balance and focus. Stand with your feet hip-width apart and shift your weight onto your left foot. Lift your right foot and place it on your left inner thigh. Press your hands together in front of your chest and hold for 30 seconds. Repeat on the other side.

2. Downward-facing dog (Adho mukha svanasana)

The downward-facing dog is a classic yoga pose that stretches the hamstrings, calves, and spine. Start on your hands and knees with your wrists directly under your shoulders and your knees under your hips. Lift your hips up and back, straightening your arms and legs. Hold for 30 seconds.

3. Warrior II (Virabhadrasana II)

The warrior II pose is a great way to improve balance and strengthen your legs. Start in a lunge position with your left foot forward. Turn your right foot out to the side and bend your left knee. Extend your arms out to the sides and gaze over your left hand. Hold for 30 seconds and repeat on the other side.

4. Cobra pose (Bhujangasana)

The cobra pose is a gentle backbend that stretches the spine and chest. Lie on your stomach with your hands under your shoulders. Press your hands into the ground and lift your chest up, keeping your elbows close to your body. Hold for 30 seconds.

5. Bridge pose (Setu bandha sarvangasana)

The bridge pose is a great way to stretch the hips and lower back. Lie on your back with your knees bent and your feet flat on the ground. Lift your hips up, keeping your feet and shoulders on the ground. Hold for 30 seconds.

In conclusion, these yoga poses are a great way for seniors to improve their flexibility and balance. They are gentle and low-impact, making them perfect for those who want to stay active as they age. Practice these poses regularly and you will notice a significant improvement in your flexibility and balance.

9.3. Yoga Poses for Strength and Endurance

Yoga poses for strength and endurance are an excellent way for seniors to maintain their physical health and overall wellbeing. These poses help seniors to improve their muscle strength, endurance, balance, and flexibility, which are essential factors for aging actively and gracefully.

The following are some of the best yoga poses for seniors to build strength and endurance:

1. Warrior I Pose: This pose strengthens the legs, hips, and core muscles. It also improves balance and concentration. To do this pose, stand with your feet hip-width apart and step your right foot back. Bend your left knee and inhale your arms overhead. Hold for five breaths and repeat on the other side.

2. Chair Pose: This pose strengthens the legs, hips, and back muscles. It also improves posture and balance. To do this pose, stand with your feet hip-width apart and inhale your arms overhead. Bend your knees and lower your hips as if you are sitting in an imaginary chair. Hold for five breaths.

3. Downward-Facing Dog Pose: This pose strengthens the arms, shoulders, and back muscles. It also improves flexibility in the hamstrings and calves. To do this pose, start on your hands and knees. Lift your hips up and back, coming into an inverted V-shape. Press your hands and feet into the ground and hold for five breaths.

4. Tree Pose: This pose strengthens the legs, hips, and core muscles. It also improves balance and concentration. To do this pose, stand with your feet hip-width apart and shift your weight onto your left foot. Bring your right foot to rest on your left inner thigh. Inhale your arms overhead and hold for five breaths. Repeat on the other side.

5. Plank Pose: This pose strengthens the arms, shoulders, and core muscles. It also improves posture and balance. To do this pose, start on your hands and knees. Step your feet back and come into a high push-up position. Keep your body in a straight line and hold for five breaths.

In conclusion, incorporating yoga poses for strength and endurance into your exercise routine can significantly improve your physical health and overall well-being. These poses are low-impact and can be modified to suit any fitness level. Remember to listen to your body and take breaks as needed. With regular practice, you will notice significant improvements in your strength, endurance, and balance.

9.4. How to Progress with Yoga Exercises

Yoga exercises for seniors are an excellent way to regain flexibility, balance, and strength without putting too much strain on your body. In this chapter, we will take a look at some tips for progressing with your yoga practice.

Firstly, it is important to remember that yoga is a journey, not a destination. You should aim to progress at your own pace and not compare yourself to others. With consistent practice, you will gradually improve your physical abilities and deepen your understanding of the practice.

When starting out with yoga, it is recommended to take beginner classes or start with gentle yoga poses. This will help you to become familiar with the basic poses and build a foundation for your practice. As you become more comfortable with the poses, you can gradually increase the intensity and duration of your sessions.

It is also important to listen to your body and avoid pushing yourself too hard. If you experience pain or discomfort during a pose, ease off and modify the pose to suit your abilities. Remember that yoga is not about pushing yourself to the limit, but rather about finding balance and harmony within your body and mind.

One way to progress with your yoga practice is to incorporate props such as blocks, straps, and blankets. These props can help you to achieve proper alignment and deepen your stretches. For example, using a block under your hand can help you to reach the floor in a forward bend without straining your back.

Finally, it is important to maintain a regular yoga practice to see progress. Even if you only have a few minutes each day, practicing yoga consistently will help you to build strength and flexibility over time.

In conclusion, yoga is a wonderful practice for seniors to improve their physical and mental health. By taking it slow, listening to your body, using props, and maintaining a regular practice, you can progress with your yoga practice and reap the many benefits it has to offer.

10. Conclusion

10.1. Recap of the Benefits of Exercise for Seniors

As we age, staying active becomes an essential part of maintaining a healthy lifestyle. Exercise has numerous benefits for seniors, including physical, mental, and emotional health. Let's recap the benefits of exercise for seniors.

Physical Benefits

Regular exercise can improve strength, balance, and flexibility, which are essential for maintaining independence as we age. Strength training exercises can help build muscle mass and improve bone density, reducing the risk of falls and fractures. Balance exercises can also help prevent falls by improving stability and coordination.

Low-impact cardio exercises such as walking, cycling, and swimming can improve cardiovascular health, lowering the risk of heart disease and stroke. Water aerobics exercises are particularly beneficial for seniors as they are low impact and reduce the strain on joints.

Stretching exercises can improve flexibility and range of motion, reducing the risk of injury and improving posture. Chair exercises for seniors are a great way to get started and improve mobility.

Mental Benefits

Exercise has been shown to improve cognitive function and reduce the risk of dementia and Alzheimer's disease. Regular exercise can also improve mood and reduce symptoms of depression and anxiety.

Emotional Benefits

Exercise can provide a sense of accomplishment and boost self-esteem. It can also provide a sense of community and socialization, particularly in group exercise classes such as yoga.

In conclusion, regular exercise is essential for seniors for physical, mental, and emotional health. Whether it's chair exercises, balance exercises, strength training, low-impact cardio, stretching, water aerobics, or yoga, there are plenty of options to choose from. Remember to consult with a doctor before starting any exercise program and start slowly, gradually increasing intensity and duration over time.

10.2. Encouragement to Continue an Active Lifestyle

As we age, it can be tempting to slow down and take things easier. However, maintaining an active lifestyle is crucial for your physical and mental health. Regular exercise can help you maintain your balance, strength, flexibility, and cardiovascular health, reducing the risk of falls, chronic disease, and cognitive decline. It can also boost your mood, energy levels, and overall quality of life.

If you're not used to exercising regularly, it's never too late to start. You don't need to run a marathon or lift heavy weights to reap the benefits of physical activity. There are plenty of exercises and activities that are safe, enjoyable, and effective for seniors of all fitness levels and abilities.

Chair exercises are a great option for seniors who might have limited mobility or balance issues. These exercises can be done while sitting in a chair or using it for support. They can help strengthen your upper body, core, and legs, as well as improve your range of motion and flexibility.

Balance exercises are also essential for seniors, as they can help prevent falls and improve your overall stability. Simple exercises like standing on one leg, walking heel to toe, or using a balance board can make a big difference in your balance and coordination.

Strength training exercises are vital for maintaining muscle mass and bone density, which can decline with age. You don't need to lift heavy weights to build strength; bodyweight exercises like squats, lunges, push-ups, and planks can be just as effective. Resistance bands and light weights can also be used to increase the challenge.

Low-impact cardio exercises like walking, swimming, or cycling are ideal for seniors who want to improve their cardiovascular health without putting too much stress on their joints. These exercises can help improve your endurance, reduce your risk of heart disease, and boost your mood.

Stretching exercises are essential for maintaining your flexibility and range of motion. Gentle stretches like neck rolls, shoulder shrugs, and hamstring stretches can help reduce tension, improve circulation, and prevent injuries.

Water aerobics exercises are a great option for seniors who want a low-impact, full-body workout. Exercising in water can reduce the impact on your joints while providing resistance and support. Activities like water walking, jogging, and aerobics can improve your cardiovascular health, build strength, and enhance your flexibility.

Yoga exercises are another great way to improve your strength, flexibility, balance, and mental health. Yoga can help reduce stress, anxiety, and depression, while improving your overall sense of wellbeing. There are many yoga poses that can be adapted for seniors, including chair yoga and gentle flows.

Whatever type of exercise you choose, it's important to listen to your body and start slowly. Aim for at least 30 minutes of moderate activity most days of the week, and mix up your routine to keep things interesting and challenging. With consistent effort and a positive attitude, you can continue an active, healthy lifestyle well into your golden years.

10.3. Additional Resources for Seniors to Stay Active

Staying active is essential for seniors to maintain a healthy lifestyle. Exercise not only helps improve physical health but also enhances mental well-being. Here are some additional resources for seniors to stay active and live an active aging lifestyle.

1. Senior centers

Senior centers are a great place to meet other seniors and partake in various activities. Many senior centers offer exercise classes, such as yoga, water aerobics, and dance classes. These classes are a great way to socialize and stay active.

2. Parks and recreation centers

Parks and recreation centers offer a variety of classes and activities for seniors. From hiking to swimming, these centers provide a great opportunity for seniors to stay active and enjoy the outdoors.

3. Online exercise programs

For seniors who prefer to exercise from the comfort of their own home, there are many online exercise programs available. These programs offer a variety of exercises, including chair exercises, stretching, and strength training exercises.

4. Fitness apps

Fitness apps are another great resource for seniors to stay active. Many of these apps offer low-impact cardio exercises, which are perfect for seniors with joint pain or mobility issues. These apps also offer tracking features, which can help seniors stay motivated and track their progress.

5. Community centers

Community centers offer a variety of activities, including exercise classes and social events. These centers are a great place for seniors to meet other seniors and stay active.

6. Silver Sneakers

Silver Sneakers is a free fitness program for seniors that is offered through many Medicare Advantage plans. The program provides seniors with access to gyms, fitness classes, and other wellness resources.

In conclusion, staying active is essential for seniors to maintain a healthy lifestyle. The above resources offer a variety of options for seniors to stay active and live an active aging lifestyle. Whether it's at a senior center, park, or online, there are many opportunities for seniors to exercise and stay healthy.

10.4 Thank You!

I would like to express my gratitude to you for taking the time to read my book. I truly hope that it has provided you with valuable insights and knowledge that you can use to succeed in your endeavors.

Additionally, I was wondering if you could do me a favor. If you found the book helpful, would you be willing to share your thoughts by leaving an honest review where you bought my book? Your reviews are incredibly important to me, and I read each and every one of them. Your support is greatly appreciated.

Thank you once again for your generous support.

Best regards,

Bolakale Aremu
Ojula Technology Innovations
OjulaTech@gmail.com

www.ingramcontent.com/pod-product-compliance
Lightning Source LLC
Chambersburg PA
CBHW012309240726
48656CB00008B/2625